Juicing for Cold and Flu:

Boost Your Immunity and Beat Cold and Flu with the Power of Juicing

Amber Denise

Table of Contents

Chapter 3: Delicious Juicing Recipes to Fight Cold and Flu

3.1 Immune-Boosting Green Juice

Classic Green Juice

Sweet and Tart Green Juice

Tropical Green Juice

Minty Green Juice

Ginger-Turmeric Green Juice

Pineapple-Carrot Green Juice

Berry Green Juice

Grapefruit Green Juice

Celery-Cucumber Green Juice

Beet-Ginger Green Juice

Cilantro-Lime Green Juice

Spicy Green Juice

Green Energy Juice:

Lemon-Ginger Green Juice

Lemon and Kale Juice

Citrusy Green Juice

Pineapple and Cilantro Juice

Green Goddess Juice

Turmeric and Beet Juice

Broccoli and Apple Juice

Ginger and Orange Juice

Fennel and Kale Juice

Parsnip and Apple Juice

3.2 Flu Fighter Juice

Super Antioxidant Juice

Flu Fighter Tonic Juice

Vitamin C Powerhouse Juice

Superfood Juice

Ginger Zinger Juice

Beet-Apple-Carrot Juice

Spiced Apple-Carrot Juice

Green Ginger Juice

Carrot, Ginger, and Turmeric Juice

Beetroot, Carrot, and Ginger Juice

Pineapple and Ginger Juice

Apple, Carrot, and Orange Juice

Red Pepper and Tomato Juice

Lemon and Honey Juice

Berry Blast Juice

Spinach, Carrot, and Orange Juice

Mango and Turmeric Juice

Cucumber and Mint Juice

Kale, Apple, and Lemon Juice

Watermelon and Lime Juice

Spicy Citrus Juice

3.3 Vitamin C Blast Juice

Classic Citrus Blast

Green C Booster

Berry Citrus Zinger

Pineapple Mango Delight

Carrot Orange Glow

Tropical Sunshine

Red Grapefruit Refresher

Minty Melon Madness

Lemon Ginger Power

Spicy Citrus Kick

3.4 Cold and Flu Buster Juice

Cold Fighter Juice

Flu Remedy Juice

Antioxidant Blast Juice

Ginger-Turmeric Immunity Boost Juice

Vitamin C Powerhouse Juice

Super Green Juice

Cold and Flu Tonic Juice

Immune-Boosting Green Juice

Chapter 4: Juicing for Prevention: How to Stay Healthy During Cold and Flu Season

Chapter 5: Juicing for Recovery: How to Get Back on Your Feet Faster

5.2 Nutrient-Dense Juices to Support Your Recovery

5.3 Foods to Avoid While Recovering

Conclusion: The Power of Juicing for Cold and Flu and Your Overall Health

INTRODUCTION

UNDERSTANDING THE BENEFITS OF JUICING FOR COLD AND FLU

Juicing is a popular method of extracting nutrients from fruits and vegetables. Many people turn to juicing as a way to boost their immune system and fight off cold and flu symptoms. the benefits of juicing for cold and flu, and how it can help you stay healthy.

Juicing has become increasingly popular as a natural remedy for cold and flu symptoms. The process of juicing involves extracting the liquid from fruits and vegetables to create a nutrient-dense drink that can help boost the immune system and promote healing.

Juicing has been around for decades as a way to incorporate fruits and vegetables into our diets in an easy and convenient way. However, what many people may not know is that juicing can also be an effective way to combat cold and flu symptoms.

Boosts immune system: Juicing is a great way to give your immune system a boost. Fruits and vegetables are packed with essential vitamins and minerals that can help strengthen your immune system, making it better equipped to fight off cold and flu viruses.

Provides hydration: When you are sick, it is important to stay hydrated. Juicing is a great way to get fluids into your body (drinking plenty of fluids can help loosen congestion and prevent dehydration) and it also provides important nutrients that can help you recover more quickly.

Reduces inflammation: Many fruits and vegetables contain anti-inflammatory properties that can help reduce inflammation in your body. When you have a cold or flu, your body may be inflamed, causing symptoms such as congestion and sore throat. Drinking juices that are high in anti-inflammatory properties can help alleviate these symptoms. In addition to ginger, other anti-inflammatory foods that are good for juicing include turmeric, pineapple, and berries.

Provides antioxidants: Fruits and vegetables are also rich in antioxidants, which can help protect your body against the damaging effects of free radicals. Free radicals can cause cellular damage and may contribute to the development of various diseases, including colds and flu. Drinking juices that are high in antioxidants can help protect your body against these harmful compounds.

Relieves symptoms: Certain fruits and vegetables contain compounds that can help relieve specific cold and flu symptoms. For example, ginger can help relieve nausea and vomiting, while garlic can help boost your immune system and reduce congestion.

Provides energy: When you are sick, you may feel weak and lethargic. Drinking fresh juices can provide you with the energy you need to get through the day. Juices are also easily digestible, which means that your body can absorb the nutrients quickly, providing you with a quick energy boost.

Improves digestion: Juicing can also improve your digestion, which is important when you are sick. Many fruits and vegetables such as apples and celery contain digestive enzymes that can help break down food and improve nutrient absorption. When your body is better able to absorb nutrients, it can more effectively fight off cold and flu viruses.

CHAPTER 1

THE IMMUNE SYSTEM: HOW IT WORKS AND HOW JUICING CAN HELP

1.1 The Basics of Immune System

The immune system is a complex network of cells, tissues, and organs that work together to protect the body from harmful substances and invaders, such as viruses, bacteria, fungi, and parasites. Its primary function is to identify and destroy foreign pathogens while leaving healthy cells and tissues intact.

There are two main types of immune responses: innate and adaptive. Innate immunity is the first line of defense against pathogens and is composed of cells and proteins that are always present in the body. These cells include natural killer cells, macrophages, and neutrophils, which can quickly identify and destroy foreign substances without prior exposure. Innate immunity also includes physical barriers such as skin and mucous membranes, which prevent pathogens from entering the body.

Adaptive immunity, on the other hand, develops over time in response to exposure to specific pathogens. It involves the activation of specialized cells called lymphocytes, which include B cells and T cells. B cells produce antibodies that can bind to and neutralize specific pathogens, while T cells can recognize and destroy infected cells. Adaptive immunity also involves the development of memory cells, which can quickly recognize and respond to specific pathogens in future exposures, resulting in a faster and more effective immune response.

The immune system also involves several organs and tissues, including the thymus, bone marrow, lymph nodes, and spleen. The thymus is responsible for the development and maturation of T cells, while the bone marrow produces all types of blood cells, including lymphocytes. Lymph nodes and the spleen are specialized tissues that filter the blood and remove foreign substances, allowing immune cells to identify and destroy them.

Overall, the immune system is an intricate and

essential defense mechanism that protects the body from harm. Understanding the basics of the immune system can help individuals make informed decisions about their health, such as taking steps to boost their immunity or seeking medical attention when necessary.

1.2 The Role of Vitamins and Nutrients in Immune System

The immune system is a complex network of cells, tissues, and organs that work together to protect the body from harmful pathogens, such as viruses, bacteria, and fungi. A healthy immune system is essential for overall health and wellbeing, and several vitamins and nutrients play a crucial role in supporting and strengthening the immune system.

Vitamin C:

Vitamin C is a powerful antioxidant that helps protect the body against harmful free radicals. It is also essential for the production of white blood cells, which are the immune system's primary defense against infections. Studies have shown that vitamin C can reduce the duration and severity of respiratory infections, such as the common cold, by boosting the immune system.

Good dietary sources of vitamin C include citrus fruits, strawberries, kiwi fruit, bell peppers, broccoli, and tomatoes.

Vitamin D:

Vitamin D is essential for bone health, but it also plays an important role in the immune system. Research has shown that vitamin D helps regulate immune function by promoting the production of antimicrobial peptides that kill harmful bacteria and viruses.

Vitamin D deficiency has been linked to an increased risk of respiratory infections, such as the flu and pneumonia. Good sources of vitamin D include fatty fish, such as salmon and tuna, fortified dairy products, and egg yolks. Sunlight is also a natural source of vitamin D.

Zinc:

Zinc is an essential mineral that plays a critical role in immune function. It is required for the development and function of white blood cells, which are the immune system's primary defense against infections. Zinc also has anti-inflammatory properties that can help reduce inflammation in the body.

Studies have shown that zinc supplements can reduce the severity and duration of colds and other respiratory infections. Good dietary sources of zinc include oysters, beef, pork, chicken, beans, and nuts.

Vitamin A:

Vitamin A is essential for vision, but it also plays an important role in the immune system. It helps maintain the integrity of the skin and mucous membranes, which are the body's first line of defense against infections.

Vitamin A also promotes the production of white blood cells, which are essential for fighting infections. Good dietary sources of vitamin A include liver, fish, eggs, and dairy products.

Vitamin E:

Vitamin E is a powerful antioxidant that helps protect the body against harmful free radicals. It also plays a role in immune function by promoting the production of white blood cells and improving their function.

Vitamin E supplements can improve immune function in older adults and people with weakened immune systems. Good dietary sources of vitamin E include nuts, seeds, vegetable oils, and leafy green vegetables.

Selenium:

Selenium is a mineral that plays an important role in immune function. It helps the body produce glutathione, a powerful antioxidant that protects the body against harmful free radicals. Selenium also promotes the production of white blood cells, which are essential for fighting infections.

Selenium supplements can improve immune function and reduce the risk of viral infections. Good dietary sources of selenium include Brazil nuts, tuna, shrimp, and whole grains.

1.3 The Benefits of Juicing for Immune System

Juicing is a popular method of extracting nutrients from fruits and vegetables to make delicious and nutritious drinks. It is an excellent way to boost your immune system by providing your body with essential vitamins, minerals, and antioxidants. In this article, we will discuss the benefits of juicing for the immune system and how it can improve your overall health.

Boosts Nutrient Intake:

Juicing is an effective way to consume a variety of fruits and vegetables that you might not normally eat. By juicing, you can obtain essential nutrients, such as vitamin C, vitamin A, and potassium, which are important for a healthy immune system. Additionally, juicing can help you reach your daily recommended intake of fruits and vegetables, which is typically five servings per day.

Increases Antioxidant Intake:

Antioxidants are compounds that protect cells from damage caused by free radicals, which are unstable molecules that can harm cells and contribute to chronic diseases. Fruits and vegetables are rich in antioxidants and juicing them can help you obtain a high concentration of antioxidants in one drink. Antioxidants such as vitamin C, vitamin E, and beta-carotene can help boost your immune system by reducing inflammation and fighting off harmful pathogens.

Improves Digestive Health:

Juicing can also help improve your digestive health, which is crucial for a healthy immune system. By removing the fiber from fruits and vegetables, juicing allows for easier absorption of nutrients, which can improve digestion and reduce inflammation. Additionally, juicing can help maintain a healthy gut microbiome by providing your body with prebiotics and probiotics, which are essential for a healthy gut.

Boosts Energy:

Juicing can help boost your energy levels, which is important for a healthy immune system. By consuming a variety of fruits and vegetables, you can obtain essential nutrients, such as vitamin B6 and magnesium, which are crucial for energy production. Additionally, the natural sugars in fruits and vegetables can provide a quick boost of energy without the crash associated with processed sugars.

Supports Overall Health:

Juicing can provide many health benefits beyond just boosting your immune system. It can help maintain a healthy weight, reduce inflammation, improve cardiovascular health, and even reduce the risk of chronic diseases such as cancer and diabetes. By consuming a variety of fruits and vegetables through juicing, you can support your overall health and well-being.

CHAPTER 2

THE BEST JUICING INGREDIENTS FOR COLD AND FLU

2.1 Fruits and Vegetables that are Rich in Vitamin C

Vitamin C, also known as ascorbic acid, is a water-soluble vitamin that is essential for various bodily functions. It plays a crucial role in maintaining the immune system, aiding in the absorption of iron, promoting the growth and repair of tissues, and acting as an antioxidant that helps protect cells from damage caused by harmful molecules known as free radicals.

While most animals can produce their own vitamin C, humans are one of the few species that cannot. Therefore, it is important to obtain sufficient amounts of this nutrient through a balanced diet that includes fruits and vegetables that are rich in vitamin C.

Here are some of the best fruits and vegetables that are excellent sources of vitamin C:

Citrus fruits: Oranges, grapefruits, lemons, limes, and tangerines are all excellent sources of vitamin C. Just one medium-sized orange contains about 70mg of vitamin C, which is more than the recommended daily intake for adults.

Berries: Strawberries, raspberries, blueberries, and blackberries are all rich in vitamin C. For example, one cup of strawberries contains about 85mg of vitamin C.

Kiwi: This small, fuzzy fruit is packed with vitamin C, with one medium-sized kiwi containing about 70mg of vitamin C.

Papaya: This tropical fruit is not only delicious but also rich in vitamin C. Just one medium-sized papaya contains about 95mg of vitamin C.

Pineapple: This tropical fruit is also a great source of vitamin C, with one cup of fresh pineapple chunks containing about 80mg of vitamin C.

Mango: This sweet and juicy fruit is also a good source of vitamin C, with one medium-sized mango containing about 60mg of vitamin C.

Guava: This tropical fruit has a unique flavor and is also a great source of vitamin C. One medium-sized guava contains about 125mg of vitamin C, which is more than the recommended daily intake for adults.

Bell peppers: Red, yellow, and green bell peppers are all excellent sources of vitamin C. Just one medium-sized red bell pepper contains about 150mg of vitamin C, which is more than twice the recommended daily intake for adults.

Broccoli: This cruciferous vegetable is not only a great source of fiber but also rich in vitamin C. One cup of chopped raw broccoli contains about 81mg of vitamin C.

Brussels sprouts: These small, cruciferous vegetables are packed with vitamin C, with one cup of cooked Brussels sprouts containing about 96mg of vitamin C.

2.2 Anti-inflammatory Ingredients to Combat Cold and Flu Symptoms

When we catch a cold or the flu, our immune system responds by triggering an inflammatory response to fight off the virus or bacteria. While this response is necessary to fight off the infection, it can also lead to uncomfortable symptoms such as fever, cough, and congestion. Anti-inflammatory ingredients can help to reduce these symptoms by calming down the immune system and reducing inflammation.

Here are some anti-inflammatory ingredients that can help combat cold and flu symptoms:

Ginger: Ginger is a natural anti-inflammatory and has been used for centuries to treat a variety of ailments. It contains compounds called gingerols and shogaols, which have been shown to reduce inflammation and pain. Ginger can help to soothe a sore throat, reduce fever, and relieve cough and congestion.

Turmeric: Turmeric is another natural anti-inflammatory that has been used in traditional medicine for centuries. It contains a compound called curcumin, which has been shown to have potent anti-inflammatory effects. Turmeric can help to reduce fever, relieve cough and congestion, and soothe a sore throat.

Garlic: Garlic is a potent natural anti-inflammatory and has been shown to have antimicrobial properties that can help fight off infections. It contains compounds called allicin and alliin, which have been shown to reduce inflammation and boost the immune system. Garlic can help to relieve cough and congestion, reduce fever, and soothe a sore throat.

Echinacea: Echinacea is an herb that has been traditionally used to treat cold and flu symptoms. It contains compounds that have been shown to have anti-inflammatory and immunomodulatory effects, meaning they can help to regulate the immune system and reduce inflammation. Echinacea can help to reduce fever, relieve cough and congestion, and boost the immune system.

Honey: Honey is a natural anti-inflammatory and has been shown to have antimicrobial properties that can help fight off infections. It can help to soothe a sore throat, reduce cough and congestion, and boost the immune system. Honey can be added to tea or warm water to help alleviate cold and flu symptoms.

Vitamin C: Vitamin C is a powerful antioxidant and has been shown to have anti-inflammatory effects. It can help to boost the immune system and reduce the severity and duration of cold and flu symptoms. Vitamin C can be found in a variety of foods such as citrus fruits, kiwi, strawberries, and bell peppers.

Omega-3 Fatty Acids: Omega-3 fatty acids are anti-inflammatory and have been shown to have immunomodulatory effects. They can help to reduce inflammation and boost the immune system, making them beneficial for combating cold and flu symptoms. Omega-3 fatty acids can be found in fatty fish such as salmon and sardines, as well as in nuts and seeds such as chia seeds and flaxseeds.

Green Tea: Green tea is a natural anti-inflammatory and has been shown to have antimicrobial properties that can help fight off infections. It contains compounds called catechins, which have been shown to reduce inflammation and boost the immune system. Green tea can help to relieve cough and congestion, reduce fever, and soothe a sore throat.

Probiotics: Probiotics are beneficial bacteria that can help to boost the immune system and reduce inflammation. They can help to prevent and treat cold and flu symptoms by improving gut health and supporting the immune system. Probiotics can be found in fermented foods such as yogurt, kefir, and sauerkraut.

2.3 Herbs and Spices for Immunity Boosting

Herbs and spices have been used for centuries to promote good health and to ward off illnesses. Many herbs and spices contain potent antioxidant, anti-inflammatory, and antimicrobial properties that can help to boost the immune system and promote overall wellness. Here are some of the best herbs and spices for immunity boosting and discuss their benefits.

Turmeric

Turmeric is a spice that has been used in Ayurvedic medicine for centuries. It contains a powerful antioxidant compound called curcumin, which has anti-inflammatory properties and can help to support the immune system. Curcumin has been shown to reduce inflammation and improve immune function by modulating the activity of immune cells. Additionally, turmeric may help to reduce the risk of chronic diseases such as heart disease, Alzheimer's, and cancer.

Garlic

Garlic is a common culinary herb that has been used for medicinal purposes for thousands of years. It contains sulfur compounds such as allicin, which have antimicrobial and antioxidant properties. Garlic has been shown to stimulate the immune system by increasing the production of white blood cells, which are essential for fighting off infections.

It may also help to reduce the risk of chronic diseases such as heart disease and cancer.

Ginger

Ginger is a root that has been used in traditional medicine for centuries. It contains a compound called gingerol, which has potent anti-inflammatory and antioxidant properties. Ginger has been shown to improve immune function by reducing inflammation and enhancing the activity of immune cells. Additionally, it may help to alleviate symptoms of respiratory infections such as cough and sore throat.

Cinnamon

Cinnamon is a spice that is commonly used in baking and cooking. It contains compounds called cinnamaldehyde and eugenol, which have antimicrobial and anti-inflammatory properties. Cinnamon has been shown to improve immune function by stimulating the production of white blood cells and enhancing the activity of immune cells. Additionally, it may help to regulate blood sugar levels and reduce the risk of chronic diseases such as diabetes and heart disease.

Echinacea

Echinacea is a herb that has been used in traditional medicine for centuries. It contains compounds called alkyl amides and polysaccharides, which have immunomodulatory properties. Echinacea has been shown to improve immune function by stimulating the activity of immune cells and enhancing the production of antibodies. Additionally, it may help to reduce the duration and severity of colds and other respiratory infections.

Oregano

Oregano is a herb that is commonly used in Mediterranean cuisine. It contains compounds called carvacrol and thymol, which have antimicrobial and antioxidant properties. Oregano has been shown to improve immune function by enhancing the activity of immune cells and reducing inflammation. Additionally, it may help to alleviate symptoms of respiratory infections such as cough and sore throat.

Rosemary

Rosemary is a herb that is commonly used in Mediterranean cuisine. It contains compounds called rosmarinic acid and carnosic acid, which have antioxidant and anti-inflammatory properties. Rosemary has been shown to improve immune function by enhancing the activity of immune cells and reducing inflammation. Additionally, it may help to improve cognitive function and reduce the risk of chronic diseases such as Alzheimer's.

Thyme

Thyme is an herb that is commonly used in Mediterranean and Middle Eastern cuisine. It contains compounds called thymol and carvacrol, which have antimicrobial and antioxidant properties. Thyme has been shown to improve immune function by enhancing the activity of immune cells and reducing inflammation. Additionally, it may help to alleviate symptoms of respiratory infections such as cough and sore throat.

CHAPTER 3

DELICIOUS JUICING RECIPES TO FIGHT COLD AND FLU

3.1 Immune-Boosting Green Juice

Here are 24 immune-boosting green juice recipes

1. Classic Green Juice:

Ingredients:

- 2 cups spinach leaves

- 1 cucumber

- 1 green apple

- 1 lemon

- 1-inch piece of ginger

- 1 celery stalk

Instructions:

1. Wash all the vegetables and fruits thoroughly.

2. Cut the cucumber, green apple, and celery into small pieces.

3. Peel the ginger and cut it into small pieces.

4. Cut the lemon in half and squeeze out the juice.

5. Add all the ingredients to a blender and blend until smooth.

6. If the consistency is too thick, add a small amount of water to thin it out.

7. Once blended, pour the juice into a glass and serve immediately.

Note: You can adjust the sweetness and tanginess of the juice by adding more or less lemon juice. You can also add other green vegetables such as kale or parsley to the recipe to enhance the nutritional value.

2. Sweet and Tart Green Juice:

- 1 green apple
- 1/2 cucumber
- 1/2 lemon
- 1/2 lime
- 1 handful of spinach
- 1 handful of kale
- 1 inch of ginger

Instructions:

1. Wash all of the ingredients thoroughly.
2. Cut the apple and cucumber into small pieces.
3. Juice the apple, cucumber, lemon, and lime.
4. Add the spinach, kale, and ginger to the juicer and juice them.
5. Mix the two juices together and stir well.
6. Pour into a glass and serve immediately.

Enjoy your sweet and tart green juice!

3. Tropical Green Juice:

- 1 cup pineapple chunks

- 1 medium banana

- 1 cup spinach leaves

- 1/2 cup coconut water

- 1/2 cup water

- 1 tsp honey (optional)

Instructions:

1. Prepare the ingredients by washing the spinach leaves, peeling the banana, and cutting the pineapple into small chunks.

2. Add the pineapple chunks, banana, and spinach leaves to a blender.

3. Pour in the coconut water and water and blend the mixture until smooth.

4. If desired, add honey to sweeten the juice.

Pour the juice into a glass and enjoy!

4. Minty Green Juice:

Ingredients:

1 large cucumber

2 cups spinach leaves

1/2 cup fresh mint leaves

2 green apples

1 lime, juiced

Instructions:

Wash all the produce well.

Peel the cucumber and cut it into chunks.

Core the apples and cut them into chunks.

Put the cucumber, spinach, mint leaves, and apple chunks into a juicer and process until smooth.

Squeeze the lime juice into the juicer and mix well.

Pour the juice into a glass and serve immediately.

Enjoy your refreshing minty green juice!

5. Ginger-Turmeric Green Juice:

Ingredients:

1 green apple, cored and chopped

2 stalks celery, chopped

1 cucumber, peeled and chopped

1-inch piece of ginger, peeled and chopped

1-inch piece of turmeric, peeled and chopped

1 lemon, juiced

2 cups of spinach

1 cup of water

Instructions:

Rinse all the ingredients well.

Cut the green apple, celery, and cucumber into small pieces.

Peel and chop the ginger and turmeric.

Juice the lemon.

In a juicer, add the chopped green apple, celery, cucumber, ginger, and turmeric.

Add the spinach and lemon juice.

Pour in the water and mix well.

Enjoy your Ginger-Turmeric Green Juice immediately.

Note: You can adjust the amount of water depending on how thick or thin you like your juice. You can also add more lemon juice for a tangier flavor.

6. Pineapple-Carrot Green Juice:

Ingredients:

2 cups of fresh pineapple chunks

2 medium-sized carrots, peeled and chopped

1 handful of spinach leaves

1 handful of kale leaves

1-inch piece of ginger, peeled and chopped

1 lemon, juiced

Instructions:

Wash all the ingredients thoroughly.

Cut the pineapple into chunks, peel and chop the carrots, and chop the ginger into small pieces.

Juice the pineapple, carrots, spinach, kale, and ginger in a juicer.

Squeeze the lemon juice into the juicer or mix it in afterwards.

Stir well and serve immediately.

Enjoy your healthy Pineapple-Carrot Green Juice!

7. Berry Green Juice:

1 cup of mixed berries (fresh or frozen)

1 large handful of fresh spinach

1 cucumber

1 apple

1 lemon, juiced

1/2 cup of water

Instructions:

Wash all of the fruits and vegetables thoroughly.

Cut the cucumber and apple into smaller pieces so that they fit in your juicer.

Put all of the ingredients, except for the lemon juice, into a juicer.

Turn on the juicer and juice all of the ingredients together.

Squeeze the lemon juice into the juice and stir well.

Serve and Enjoy your refreshing Berry Green Juice!

8. Grapefruit Green Juice:

Ingredients:

1 grapefruit, peeled and sliced

1 large handful of spinach

1 small cucumber, sliced

1 green apple, sliced

1/2 lemon, juiced

1-inch piece of ginger, peeled

Instructions:

Wash all the fruits and vegetables thoroughly.

Peel and slice the grapefruit and add it to your juicer along with the spinach, cucumber, and green apple.

Juice the ingredients until you get a smooth liquid.

Add the lemon juice and ginger to the mixture and stir well.

Serve and enjoy!

9. Celery-Cucumber Green Juice:

Ingredients:

3-4 celery stalks

1 large cucumber

1 lemon

Handful of parsley

Optional: a small piece of ginger root or a pinch of cayenne pepper

Instructions:

Wash all the vegetables and chop them into smaller pieces that will fit into your juicer.

Juice the celery and cucumber, alternating pieces of each in the juicer to ensure they're well mixed.

Squeeze the lemon and add the juice to the celery-cucumber mix.

Add the handful of parsley to the juicer and juice it.

Optional: If you want a bit of a kick to your juice, add a small piece of ginger root or a pinch of cayenne pepper to the juicer as well.

Stir the juice and pour it into a glass.

Enjoy your refreshing and healthy celery-cucumber green juice!

Note: If you don't have a juicer, you can blend the ingredients in a high-speed blender and then strain the mixture through a fine-mesh sieve or a nut milk bag. However, the texture may be slightly different.

You can also adjust the amounts of celery, cucumber, lemon, and parsley according to your taste preferences.

10. Beet-Ginger Green Juice:

1 medium-sized beetroot, chopped into small pieces

1-inch fresh ginger root, peeled and chopped

2 cups packed baby spinach

1 medium-sized green apple, chopped into small pieces

1 medium-sized cucumber, chopped into small pieces

1 lemon, juiced

Instructions:

Wash all the vegetables thoroughly.

Chop the beetroot, ginger, apple, and cucumber into small pieces.

Add the chopped vegetables and baby spinach to a blender or juicer and blend until smooth.

Squeeze the lemon and add the juice to the mixture.

Pour the juice into a glass and serve immediately.

Enjoy your fresh and healthy Beet-Ginger Green Juice!

Note: If you prefer a sweeter taste, you can add a teaspoon of honey or maple syrup to the mixture. Also, you can adjust the quantity of ginger based on your preference.

11. Cilantro-Lime Green Juice:

Ingredients:

2 cups packed fresh cilantro

1 medium cucumber

2 limes, juiced

2 cups fresh baby spinach

1 green apple, cored and chopped

1-inch piece fresh ginger, peeled

1/4 cup water

Instructions:

Rinse the cilantro, cucumber, spinach, and apple well.

Cut the cucumber into chunks.

Add all ingredients to a blender and blend until smooth.

If the mixture is too thick, add more water until it reaches the desired consistency.

Pour into glasses and serve immediately.

Enjoy your refreshing cilantro-lime green juice!

12. Spicy Green Juice

Ingredients:

2 green apples, cored and chopped

2 cucumbers, chopped

1 handful of fresh spinach

1 handful of fresh kale

1 lemon, peeled

1-inch piece of ginger, peeled

1 jalapeño pepper, seeded and chopped

1/2 cup of water

Instructions:

Wash and prepare all the ingredients as described above.

Add all the ingredients to a high-speed blender.

Blend the mixture until smooth and all the ingredients are well combined.

If the juice is too thick, add a little more water to thin it out.

Pour the juice into a glass and enjoy immediately.

Note: If you're not a fan of spicy drinks, you can omit the jalapeño pepper or reduce the amount to your liking. You can also add a little honey or agave nectar to sweeten the juice if needed.

13. Green Energy Juice:

2 cups of fresh spinach leaves

1 green apple, cored and sliced

1 cucumber, peeled and chopped

1 lemon, juiced

1-inch piece of ginger, peeled and chopped

1 handful of fresh mint leaves

1/2 cup of water

Instructions:

Wash and prepare all of the ingredients as directed.

Add the spinach, green apple, cucumber, lemon juice, ginger, and mint leaves to a juicer.

Process the ingredients until they are all juiced.

Add the water to the juice and stir well.

Serve and Enjoy your delicious and nutritious green energy juice!

14. Lemon-Ginger Green Juice:

Ingredients:

1 cucumber

1 green apple

1 lcmon

1-inch fresh ginger root

2 cups spinach

1/2 cup water

Instructions:

Wash all the ingredients thoroughly.

Peel the lemon and ginger and cut the cucumber and apple into pieces that will fit in your juicer.

Juice the cucumber, apple, lemon, and ginger.

Add the spinach to the juicer and juice again.

Add water to the juice and mix well.

Pour the juice into a glass and enjoy!

15. Lemon and Kale Juice

Ingredients:

2 cups chopped kale

1 lemon, peeled and sliced

1 apple, chopped

1 inch piece of ginger, peeled and chopped

1/2 cup water

Instructions:

Wash the kale leaves thoroughly and remove the hard stems.

Add the kale, lemon, apple, and ginger to a blender or juicer.

Add 1/2 cup of water to the blender or juicer.

Blend or juice the ingredients until smooth.

Strain the mixture through a fine mesh strainer or cheesecloth to remove any pulp.

Serve the juice over ice and enjoy immediately.

Note: You can adjust the amount of water depending on how thick or thin you prefer your juice. You can also add a little honey or agave syrup to sweeten the juice if desired.

16. Citrusy Green Juice

Ingredients:

1 medium-sized green apple

1/2 large cucumber

1/2 lemon

1 handful of spinach

1 small piece of ginger

1/2 cup of water

Instructions:

Wash all the ingredients thoroughly.

Cut the apple and cucumber into small pieces and remove the seeds.

Squeeze the lemon juice into a blender or juicer.

Add the apple, cucumber, spinach, ginger, and water to the blender or juicer.

Blend or juice the ingredients until smooth.

Pour the juice into a glass and serve immediately.

Enjoy your refreshing citrusy green juice!

17. Pineapple and Cilantro Juice

Ingredients:

2 cups fresh pineapple chunks

1/4 cup fresh cilantro leaves

1 tablespoon lime juice

1 cup water

1 tablespoon honey (optional)

Ice cubes (optional)

Instructions:

Add the pineapple chunks, cilantro leaves, lime juice, and water to a blender.

Blend until smooth.

Taste the juice and add honey if desired.

If you want your juice to be colder, add ice cubes and blend again.

Pour the juice into glasses and serve immediately.

Enjoy your refreshing Pineapple and Cilantro Juice!

18. Green Goddess Juice

Ingredients:

1 large cucumber

1 handful of spinach

1 green apple

1 lemon

1-inch piece of ginger

1/2 cup of water (optional, for desired consistency)

Instructions:

Wash all ingredients thoroughly.

Cut the cucumber into small pieces.

Cut the apple into quarters and remove the seeds.

Peel the lemon and ginger.

Put all the ingredients into a juicer and process until smooth.

If the juice is too thick, add some water to thin it out.

Serve and enjoy!

Note: This recipe makes approximately 2 servings. Adjust the quantity of ingredients according to your desired amount of servings. Also, you can add or subtract ingredients according to your taste.

19. Turmeric and Beet Juice

Ingredients:

1 medium-sized beetroot, peeled and chopped

1 medium-sized carrot, peeled and chopped

1 small piece of ginger, peeled and chopped

1/2 teaspoon ground turmeric

1/2 lemon, juiced

1 cup water

Instructions:

Add the chopped beetroot, carrot, and ginger to a juicer and extract the juice.

Pour the juice into a glass.

Add the ground turmeric and lemon juice to the glass and stir well.

Add water to adjust the consistency to your liking.

Drink the juice immediately or refrigerate for up to 24 hours.

This juice is not only delicious, but it's also packed with nutrients such as vitamin C, potassium, and antioxidants. Enjoy!

20. Broccoli and Apple Juice

Ingredients:

1 broccoli head

2 green apples

1/2 lemon, peeled

1/2-inch piece of fresh ginger

1/2 cup of water (optional)

Instructions:

Wash the broccoli and green apples thoroughly.

Cut the broccoli into small florets and remove the stems.

Cut the apples into quarters, removing the seeds and core.

Cut the lemon into quarters, removing the peel.

Peel the ginger and slice it into thin pieces.

Add all the ingredients to a juicer or blender and blend until smooth.

If the mixture is too thick, add 1/2 cup of water to thin it out.

Pour the juice into glasses and enjoy immediately.

This juice is packed with nutrients from the broccoli and apples, while the lemon and ginger add a zesty kick. It's a great way to start your day or to enjoy as a healthy snack.

21. Ginger and Orange Juice

Ingredients:

2-3 large oranges

1-inch piece of fresh ginger

1 tablespoon honey (optional)

1 cup of water

Ice cubes (optional)

Instructions:

Peel the ginger and chop it into small pieces.

Squeeze the oranges to extract the juice and strain it to remove any seeds or pulp.

In a blender, blend the chopped ginger with water until smooth.

Strain the ginger water through a fine-mesh strainer to remove any fibers.

In a glass, combine the orange juice, ginger water, and honey (if using). Stir well to combine.

Add ice cubes and enjoy your refreshing Ginger and Orange Juice!

Note: You can adjust the amount of ginger and honey to suit your taste. You can also use a juicer instead of a blender to extract the juice from the oranges.

22. Fennel and Kale Juice

Ingredients:

1 large fennel bulb, chopped

2 cups chopped kale leaves

1 medium cucumber, chopped

2 green apples, cored and chopped

1 lemon, juiced

1-inch piece of ginger, peeled and grated

1/2 cup water

Instructions:

Wash all produce thoroughly.

Chop the fennel, kale, cucumber, and green apples into pieces that will fit in your juicer.

Juice the fennel, kale, cucumber, and green apples in your juicer, following the manufacturer's instructions.

Stir in the lemon juice, grated ginger, and water.

Pour into glasses and enjoy immediately.

Note: If you prefer a sweeter juice, you can add more apples or a small amount of honey.

23. Parsnip and Apple Juice

Ingredients:

2 medium-sized parsnips, washed and peeled

2 medium-sized apples, cored and sliced

1/2 lemon, juiced

1 inch piece of fresh ginger, peeled and chopped

1 cup of water

ice cubes (optional)

Instructions:

Cut the parsnips into small pieces so they can easily fit into your juicer. Cut the apples into slices.

Juice the parsnips, apples, and ginger in your juicer.

Squeeze the juice of half a lemon into the mixture.

Add a cup of water to the juice to dilute it slightly and stir well.

Pour the juice into glasses filled with ice cubes, if desired.

Serve immediately and enjoy!

Note: If you don't have a juicer, you can use a blender to make this recipe. Simply blend the parsnips, apples, ginger, and water until smooth, then strain the mixture through a fine mesh sieve or cheesecloth to remove any solids. Add lemon juice to taste and serve over ice (if desired)

Note: It's always best to use fresh, organic produce when making juice. And remember to wash your fruits and vegetables thoroughly before juicing them.

3.2 Flu Fighter Juice

Here are 21 immune-boosting green juice recipes

1. Super Antioxidant Juice

Ingredients:

1 cup blueberries

1 cup strawberries

1 cup raspberries

1 cup kale leaves

1 medium-sized carrot

1/2 medium-sized beetroot

1/2 lemon, juiced

1-inch piece of fresh ginger root

1-2 cups water (depending on desired consistency)

Instructions:

Wash all the fruits and vegetables thoroughly.

Cut the carrot and beetroot into small pieces.

In a juicer, blend all the fruits and vegetables until smooth.

Add the lemon juice and ginger root to the juicer and blend again.

If the juice is too thick, add water to achieve the desired consistency.

Serve chilled and enjoy!

2. Flu Fighter Tonic Juice

Ingredients:

1 orange, peeled

1 lemon, peeled

1-inch piece of ginger, peeled

1/2 teaspoon of turmeric powder

1 tablespoon of honey

1 cup of water

Instructions:

Cut the orange and lemon into small pieces and put them in a blender.

Add the peeled ginger, turmeric powder, honey, and water to the blender.

Blend all the ingredients together until you get a smooth consistency.

Strain the juice to remove any pulp or seeds.

Serve the juice in a glass and enjoy!

This juice is packed with vitamin C, antioxidants, and anti-inflammatory properties that can help boost your immune system and fight off the flu. It's a great way to start your day and keep your body healthy and strong.

3. Vitamin C Powerhouse Juice

Ingredients:

1 medium orange, peeled and sliced

1 medium grapefruit, peeled and sliced

1 lemon, peeled and sliced

1 inch piece of fresh ginger, peeled and sliced

1 medium carrot, peeled and sliced

1/2 cup of water

Instructions:

Combine all ingredients in a blender.

Blend until smooth.

If the juice is too thick, add more water to reach your desired consistency.

Pour the juice into a glass and enjoy!

This juice is high in vitamin C, which can help boost your immune system and fight off colds and flu. It also contains ginger, which has anti-inflammatory and antioxidant properties and may help alleviate nausea and sore throat. The carrot provides additional vitamins and antioxidants.

4. Superfood Juice

Ingredients:

1 medium-sized orange, peeled

1 medium-sized lemon, peeled

1 medium-sized grapefruit, peeled

1 small piece of ginger root, peeled and chopped

1 small piece of turmeric root, peeled and chopped

1 teaspoon of honey (optional)

1 cup of water

Ice cubes (optional)

Instructions:

Wash and peel the orange, lemon, and grapefruit.

Cut them into small pieces and put them in a blender.

Add the chopped ginger root and turmeric root to the blender.

Add one cup of water to the blender.

Blend all the ingredients until smooth.

If the juice is too thick, add more water.

If you want the juice to be sweeter, add a teaspoon of honey.

Pour the juice into a glass and add ice cubes if desired.

Drink the juice immediately.

This juice contains a high dose of vitamin C, which helps to boost your immune system and fight off flu viruses. Ginger and turmeric have anti-inflammatory properties that can help relieve flu symptoms like fever, sore throat, and cough.

Additionally, the honey in the juice can help soothe a sore throat.

5. Ginger Zinger Juice

Ingredients:

2 medium oranges, peeled and segmented

1 medium lemon, peeled and segmented

1 medium apple, cored and sliced

1-inch piece of fresh ginger root, peeled and sliced

1/2 cup water

Ice cubes (optional)

Instructions:

In a blender, combine the oranges, lemon, apple, ginger, and water.

Blend on high until the mixture is smooth.

If desired, add ice cubes and blend again until smooth.

Pour into glasses and enjoy immediately.

This juice is packed with vitamin C, antioxidants, and anti-inflammatory compounds that may help boost the immune system and fight off the flu. The ginger may also help reduce inflammation and soothe a sore throat.

6. Beet-Apple-Carrot Juice

Ingredients:

1 medium-sized beetroot

2 medium-sized carrots

2 medium-sized apples

1-inch piece of ginger

1 lemon (optional)

Instructions:

Wash and peel the beetroot, carrots, apples, and ginger.

Cut them into small pieces and put them in a juicer.

Turn on the juicer and process the ingredients until they are all juiced.

Squeeze the lemon (if using) into the juice and mix well.

Serve the juice immediately and enjoy.

This juice is packed with vitamins, minerals, and antioxidants that can help boost your immune system and fight off the flu. The beetroot is rich in vitamin C and iron, which are both important for a healthy immune system. Carrots are loaded with beta-carotene, which is converted to vitamin A in the body, and vitamin A helps to maintain healthy mucous membranes in the respiratory system. Apples are high in vitamin C and fiber, and ginger is a natural anti-inflammatory that can help ease symptoms of the flu.

7. Spiced Apple-Carrot Juice

Ingredients:

2 medium-sized carrots, washed and chopped

2 medium-sized apples, cored and chopped

1/2-inch fresh ginger root, peeled and chopped

1/2 teaspoon ground cinnamon

1/4 teaspoon ground nutmeg

1/4 teaspoon ground cloves

1/4 teaspoon turmeric

1 tablespoon honey (optional)

1 cup water

Instructions:

Add the chopped carrots, apples, and ginger to a blender or juicer.

Add the ground cinnamon, nutmeg, cloves, and turmeric to the blender.

Pour in the water and blend until everything is well combined and the mixture is smooth.

If you prefer a sweeter juice, add a tablespoon of honey and blend again.

Pour the juice into a glass and enjoy immediately.

This spiced apple-carrot flu fighter juice is rich in vitamins, minerals, and antioxidants that can help boost your immune system and fight off cold and flu symptoms. The carrots and apples provide a good source of vitamin C, while the ginger and spices help to reduce inflammation and ease nausea. Enjoy this delicious and healthy juice as a preventative measure or when you're feeling under the weather.

8. Green Ginger Juice

Ingredients:

1-inch piece of ginger root, peeled

1 lemon, peeled

2 green apples

2 large handfuls of spinach

1 cucumber

1/2 cup of water

Instructions:

Wash all of the produce thoroughly.

Cut the ginger, lemon, and apples into small pieces.

Cut the cucumber into slices.

Add all of the ingredients to a juicer.

Juice everything together until well combined.

Pour the juice into a glass and enjoy!

This juice is packed with vitamins, minerals, and antioxidants that can help support your immune system and keep you healthy. Ginger is known for its anti-inflammatory properties and can help soothe sore throats and reduce fever. Lemon is high in vitamin C, which is essential for a healthy immune system, and can also help improve digestion. Apples are rich in vitamins and minerals and can help reduce inflammation in the body. Spinach is loaded with antioxidants and can help support your immune system. Cucumber is a great source of hydration and can help flush out toxins from the body. Enjoy this delicious and healthy juice as part of your daily routine to help keep the flu at bay!

9. Carrot, Ginger, and Turmeric Juice

Ingredients:

2 medium-sized carrots

1 inch of ginger root

1 inch of fresh turmeric root

1/2 lemon, juiced

1/2 cup of water

Instructions:

Wash the carrots, ginger, and turmeric root.

Cut the carrots, ginger, and turmeric root into small pieces.

Put the carrot, ginger, and turmeric pieces into a blender or juicer.

Add the lemon juice and water to the blender or juicer.

Blend or juice until the ingredients are thoroughly mixed.

Pour the juice into a glass.

Enjoy your flu-fighting juice!

10. Beetroot, Carrot, and Ginger Juice

Ingredients:

1 medium-sized beetroot

2 medium-sized carrots

1-inch piece of ginger root

Water (optional)

Instructions:

Wash the beetroot, carrots, and ginger root thoroughly.

Cut the beetroot and carrots into small pieces that fit into your juicer.

Peel the ginger root and cut it into small pieces.

Add all the ingredients into a juicer and blend until you get a smooth juice.

If the juice is too thick, you can add a small amount of water to dilute it to your preferred consistency.

Pour the juice into a glass and enjoy immediately.

This juice is rich in vitamins and minerals that are essential for boosting your immune system and fighting off the flu. Beetroot is a great source of antioxidants and has anti-inflammatory properties. Carrots are loaded with vitamin A, which helps to strengthen your immune system, and ginger is known for its anti-inflammatory and antiviral properties, which can help you fight off infections. Drinking this juice regularly can help you stay healthy and fight off the flu.

11. Pineapple and Ginger Juice

Ingredients:

1 cup fresh pineapple chunks

1-inch piece of fresh ginger root

1/2 lemon

1/4 teaspoon turmeric powder (optional)

1/2 cup water

Instructions:

Peel the ginger root and cut it into small pieces.

Juice the pineapple and ginger in a juicer.

Squeeze the lemon into the juice.

Add the turmeric powder (optional) and mix well.

If the juice is too thick, add water and mix again.

Pour the juice into a glass and enjoy!

Note: If you don't have a juicer, you can blend the pineapple and ginger in a blender with the water, then strain the mixture through a fine mesh strainer to remove the pulp. Add the lemon juice and turmeric powder (if using) and mix well before serving.

12. Apple, Carrot, and Orange Juice

Ingredients:

2 medium apples, cored and sliced

2 medium carrots, peeled and chopped

1 large orange, peeled and sliced

Instructions:

Wash and prepare the fruits and vegetables.

Run all the ingredients through a juicer.

Serve the juice immediately over ice or store it in the refrigerator for up to 24 hours.

Enjoy!

13. Red Pepper and Tomato Juice

Ingredients:

2 medium-sized red bell peppers

4 medium-sized tomatoes

1 small piece of ginger (about 1 inch)

1 small lemon, juiced

1/4 teaspoon cayenne pepper (optional)

1/4 teaspoon sea salt

1/4 teaspoon black pepper

1 cup of water

Instructions:

Rinse the red bell peppers and tomatoes thoroughly, and then chop them into small pieces.

Peel the ginger and chop it into small pieces.

Place the chopped red bell peppers, tomatoes, and ginger into a blender or juicer. Add the lemon juice, cayenne pepper (if using), sea salt, black pepper, and water.

Blend or juice the mixture until smooth.

Pour the juice into a glass and serve immediately.

This red pepper and tomato juice is rich in vitamin C, antioxidants, and other immune-boosting nutrients that can help fight off colds and flu. The cayenne pepper adds a spicy kick and can also help to clear congestion. Enjoy!

14. Lemon and Honey Juice

Lemon and honey are both great natural ingredients that can help boost the immune system and fight off cold and flu viruses. Here is a simple recipe for a flu-fighting juice using these ingredients:

Ingredients:

1 lemon

1 tablespoon honey

1 cup warm water

Instructions:

Cut the lemon in half and squeeze the juice into a glass.

Add the honey to the glass.

Pour the warm water into the glass and stir the mixture until the honey is completely dissolved.

Drink the juice while it is still warm.

This lemon and honey juice can help soothe a sore throat, reduce inflammation, and boost the immune system. It is a simple and natural remedy that can be made easily at home.

15. Berry Blast Juice

Ingredients:

1 cup blueberries

1 cup strawberries

1 cup raspberries

1 orange, peeled

1 lemon, juiced

1-inch piece of ginger, peeled and grated

1 tablespoon honey

1 cup water

Instructions:

Rinse all the berries and pat them dry with a paper towel.

Peel the orange and juice the lemon.

Grate the ginger and set aside.

Add all the ingredients to a blender and blend until smooth.

If the juice is too thick, add more water to thin it out to your desired consistency.

Taste the juice and add more honey if you prefer it sweeter.

Pour the juice into a glass and enjoy immediately.

This juice is packed with antioxidants, vitamin C, and other nutrients that can help boost your immune system and fight off the flu. Drink it regularly as part of a healthy diet to stay healthy and strong.

16. Spinach, Carrot, and Orange Juice

Ingredients:

2 cups spinach leaves, washed and dried

4 medium carrots, washed and peeled

2 medium oranges, peeled and segmented

1-inch piece of fresh ginger root, peeled and grated

1 tablespoon honey (optional)

Instructions:

Wash and prepare all the ingredients.

Cut the carrots into small pieces to fit through the juicer.

Juice the spinach, carrots, oranges, and ginger through a juicer.

Stir in the honey, if desired.

Serve the juice immediately over ice(if desired) or store in a sealed container in the refrigerator for up to 24 hours.

This juice is packed with vitamins, minerals, and antioxidants that can help boost your immune system and fight off the flu. The spinach and carrots are rich in vitamin C, while the oranges provide vitamin A and potassium. Ginger is known for its anti-inflammatory properties, and honey can help soothe a sore throat. Enjoy!

17. Mango and Turmeric Juice

Mango and turmeric are both known for their immune-boosting properties, making them great ingredients for a flu-fighting juice. Herc's a recipe for a simple and delicious mango and turmeric juice:

Ingredients:

2 ripe mangoes, peeled and diced

1 teaspoon turmeric powder

1/2 lemon, juiced

1/2 teaspoon honey (optional)

1/2 cup water

Instructions:

Add the diced mangoes, turmeric powder, lemon juice, honey (if using), and water to a blender.

Blend on high speed until the mixture is smooth and creamy.

If the mixture is too thick, you can add more water to achieve your desired consistency.

Pour the juice into a glass and enjoy immediately.

This juice is not only delicious, but it's also packed with immune-boosting nutrients to help fight off the flu. The mangoes provide a healthy dose of vitamin C, while the turmeric is known for its anti-inflammatory properties. Give it a try and see how it can help you stay healthy!

18. Cucumber and Mint Juice

Cucumber and mint are both refreshing ingredients that are packed with nutrients and antioxidants that can help support the immune system. Here's a recipe:

Ingredients:

1 cucumber, peeled and chopped

1/2 cup fresh mint leaves

1 lemon, juiced

1-inch piece of ginger, peeled and grated

1/4 teaspoon cayenne pepper

1/2 cup water

Instructions:

Add the chopped cucumber and fresh mint leaves to a blender or food processor and blend until smooth.

Add the lemon juice, grated ginger, cayenne pepper, and water to the blender and blend until all ingredients are well combined.

If the mixture is too thick, add more water as needed until you reach your desired consistency.

Serve the juice immediately or store it in an airtight container in the refrigerator for up to 24 hours.

This juice is best consumed as part of a healthy and balanced diet to help support the immune system and promote overall wellness.

19. Kale, Apple, and Lemon Juice

Ingredients:

2-3 kale leaves

2 medium-sized apples

1 lemon

Instructions:

Wash the kale leaves and remove the stems.

Cut the apples into slices, removing the seeds and core.

Cut the lemon in half.

Use a juicer to extract the juice from the kale leaves, apples, and lemon.

Mix the juices well.

Serve immediately and enjoy!

Kale is a superfood that's packed with vitamins and minerals, including vitamin C, which is known to boost the immune system. Apples are also high in vitamin C, as well as antioxidants that can help fight off infection. Lemons contain vitamin C and flavonoids, which have anti-inflammatory and immune-boosting properties. Together, these ingredients make a powerful flu-fighting juice that's also delicious!

20. Watermelon and Lime Juice

Ingredients:

1 small watermelon, cubed

2 limes, juiced

1 tablespoon of honey

1/2 inch of fresh ginger, peeled and grated

1/4 teaspoon of cayenne pepper (optional)

Ice cubes (optional)

Instructions:

Cut the watermelon into small cubes and remove the seeds.

Juice the limes and set aside.

Grate the ginger and set aside.

In a blender, combine the watermelon cubes, lime juice, honey, grated ginger, and cayenne pepper (if using).

Blend until smooth.

Add ice cubes and blend again until the ice is crushed and the mixture is slushy.

Pour into glasses and serve immediately.

This juice is high in vitamin C, which can help boost your immune system and fight off cold and flu viruses. The honey and ginger also have anti-inflammatory properties, which can help reduce symptoms such as sore throat and cough. The cayenne pepper, although optional, can also help to clear your sinuses and reduce congestion. Enjoy!

21. Spicy Citrus Juice

Ingredients:

2 oranges

1 lemon

1/2-inch ginger root

1/4 tsp cayenne pepper

1 tbsp honey

1 cup water

Instructions:

Peel the oranges and lemon and cut them into small pieces.

Peel the ginger root and cut it into small pieces.

Add the oranges, lemon, ginger root, cayenne pepper, honey, and water to a blender.

Blend everything together until smooth.

Pour the juice into a glass and drink immediately.

This juice is high in vitamin C, which can help boost your immune system, and the ginger and cayenne pepper can help soothe a sore throat and alleviate congestion. It's also a great way to stay hydrated and energized when you're feeling under the weather.

3.3 Vitamin C Blast Juice

Classic Citrus Blast:

2 oranges

1 grapefruit

1 lemon

1-inch piece of ginger

1/2 cup of water

Peel and cut the oranges, grapefruit and lemon into wedges. Add them to a blender along with ginger, water. Blend until smooth and enjoy.

Green C Booster:

1 orange

1 kiwi

1/2 cup of pineapple

1/2 cup of spinach

1/2 cup of water

Peel and cut the orange and kiwi into wedges. Add them to a blender along with pineapple, spinach, water. Blend until smooth and enjoy.

Berry Citrus Zinger:

1 orange

1/2 cup of strawberries

1/2 cup of blueberries

1/2 cup of raspberries

1/2 cup of water

Ice cubes (optional)

Peel and cut the orange into wedges. Add them to a blender along with strawberries, blueberries, raspberries, water and ice. Blend until smooth and enjoy.

NB: If adding ice makes the juice too uncomfortable to drink, it's best to leave it out.

Pineapple Mango Delight:

1 cup of pineapple

1 cup of mango

1/2 cup of orange juice

1/2 cup of water

Ice cubes (optional)

Cut the pineapple and mango into chunks. Add them to a blender along with orange juice, water and ice. Blend until smooth and enjoy.

Carrot Orange Glow:

2 oranges

2 large carrots

1-inch piece of ginger

1/2 cup of water

Ice cubes (optional)

Peel and cut the oranges into wedges. Add them to a blender along with carrots, ginger, water and ice. Blend until smooth and enjoy.

Tropical Sunshine:

1 orange

1 banana

1/2 cup of pineapple

1/2 cup of mango

1/2 cup of coconut water

Ice cubes (optional)

Peel and cut the orange into wedges. Add them to a blender along with banana, pineapple, mango, coconut water and ice. Blend until smooth and enjoy.

Red Grapefruit Refresher:

1 red grapefruit

1 apple

1/2 cup of water

Ice cubes (optional)

Peel and cut the grapefruit into wedges. Core the apple and cut into chunks. Add them to a blender along with water and ice. Blend until smooth and enjoy.

Minty Melon Madness:

1 cup of honeydew melon

1 cup of watermelon

1/2 cup of fresh mint leaves

1/2 cup of water

Ice cubes (optional)

Cut the honeydew melon and watermelon into chunks. Add them to a blender along with fresh mint leaves, water and ice. Blend until smooth and enjoy.

Lemon Ginger Power:

2 lemons

1-inch piece of ginger

1 tablespoon of honey

1/2 cup of water

Ice cubes (if desired)

Peel and cut the lemons into wedges. Add them to a blender along with ginger, honey, water and ice. Blend until smooth and enjoy.

Spicy Citrus Kick:

Ingredients:

2 oranges

1 lemon

1 lime

1/2-inch ginger root, peeled

1/4 teaspoon cayenne pepper

1/4 teaspoon turmeric powder

1 cup water

Ice (if desired)

Instructions:

Peel the oranges and remove any seeds.

Cut the lemon and lime in half and squeeze out the juice, removing any seeds.

Peel the ginger root and slice it into small pieces.

Add the oranges, lemon juice, lime juice, ginger, cayenne pepper, turmeric powder, and water to a blender.

Blend until smooth.

Taste and adjust the amount of cayenne pepper and turmeric powder to your liking.

Serve over ice, if desired.

Enjoy your Spicy Citrus Kick juice! It's a refreshing and invigorating drink that's perfect for boosting your energy levels and giving you a kick of spice.

3.4 Cold and Flu Buster Juice

Here are 15 juice recipes that are packed with nutrients to help you fight off colds and flu:

1. Cold Fighter Juice

Cold Fighter Juice is a refreshing and healthy drink that is packed with nutrients to help boost your immune system and keep you feeling energized throughout the day. This juice is made from a combination of fruits and vegetables that are high in vitamins, minerals, and antioxidants, making it an excellent way to support your overall health.

The main ingredients in Cold Fighter Juice are oranges, carrots, ginger, turmeric, and lemon. Oranges are high in vitamin C, which is essential for a healthy immune system, while carrots are rich in beta-carotene, which is converted into vitamin A in the body and helps support healthy skin, eyes, and immune function.

Ginger and turmeric are both powerful anti-inflammatory ingredients that have been used for centuries in traditional medicine to help combat various ailments. They also have a warming effect on the body, which can be especially helpful during the colder months of the year when cold and flu season is in full swing.

Lemons are another excellent source of vitamin C, and they also contain other beneficial nutrients like potassium and antioxidants. They can help support healthy digestion and provide a refreshing citrusy flavor to the juice.

To make Cold Fighter Juice, you will need the following ingredients:

2 large oranges

1 lemon

1-inch piece of ginger

2 large carrots

1 medium-sized beetroot

1 tablespoon of honey (optional)

Instructions:

Peel the oranges and lemon and chop them into smaller pieces.

Peel the ginger and cut it into small chunks.

Wash the carrots and beetroot thoroughly, peel them, and cut them into smaller pieces.

Place all the ingredients, including the honey (if using), into a juicer.

Turn on the juicer and juice all the ingredients until they are well combined and the juice is smooth.

Pour the juice into a glass and serve immediately.

Cold Fighter Juice is best served chilled (also depends on personal preference), so you can refrigerate it for a few hours before serving or pour it over ice. You can also add a pinch of black pepper to the juice to enhance the absorption of turmeric, as black pepper contains piperine, which can increase the bioavailability of curcumin, the active compound in turmeric.

Enjoy!

2. Flu Remedy Juice

Flu remedy juice is a combination of several nutrient-rich ingredients that can help boost the immune system and reduce inflammation.

Flu remedy juice typically contains ingredients such as ginger, lemon, turmeric, honey, and cayenne pepper, all of which are known for their anti-inflammatory and immune-boosting properties. Ginger, for instance, contains compounds that have been shown to help reduce inflammation in the body, while lemon is high in vitamin C, which is essential for immune function. Turmeric contains curcumin, a potent anti-inflammatory compound that has been shown to help reduce pain and inflammation, while honey has antibacterial and antiviral properties. Cayenne pepper is also rich in vitamin C and contains capsaicin, a compound that can help clear sinuses and relieve congestion.

To make flu remedy juice, you will need the following ingredients:

1-2 inches of fresh ginger root

1 lemon, juiced

1-2 teaspoons of turmeric powder

1-2 tablespoons of honey

A pinch of cayenne pepper

2-3 cups of filtered water

Instructions:

Peel and chop the ginger into small pieces.

In a blender, combine the chopped ginger, lemon juice, turmeric powder, honey, cayenne pepper, and water.

Blend on high until the mixture is smooth and well-combined.

Strain the juice through a fine-mesh strainer or cheesecloth to remove any pulp or solids.

Serve the juice immediately, either chilled or at room temperature.

3. Antioxidant Blast Juice

Antioxidant Blast Cold and Flu Juice is a healthy and tasty drink that can help boost your immune system and ward off cold and flu symptoms. Here's a simple recipe for making this juice:

Ingredients:

2 medium-sized oranges, peeled

1 cup of frozen or fresh mixed berries (such as blueberries, raspberries, and strawberries)

1 small piece of ginger, peeled

1 medium-sized carrot, peeled and chopped

1/2 cup of water

Instructions:

Add all the ingredients to a blender and blend until smooth.

Pour the juice into a glass and enjoy immediately.

This juice is packed with immune-boosting

nutrients, including vitamin C from the oranges, antioxidants from the berries, and anti-inflammatory compounds from the ginger. The carrot adds an extra boost of beta-carotene, which is converted to vitamin A in the body and helps support the immune system. The water helps to thin out the juice and make it easier to blend. Enjoy this refreshing and healthy juice as part of your daily routine during cold and flu season, or anytime you want a delicious and nutritious boost!

4. Ginger-Turmeric Immunity Boost Juice

Ginger-Turmeric Immunity Boost Juice is a great way to boost your immune system and improve your overall health. Here's a simple recipe you can try at home:

Ingredients:

1 large piece of ginger

1 large piece of turmeric

1 lemon

1-2 teaspoons of honey (optional)

2-3 cups of water

Instructions:

Peel and chop the ginger and turmeric into small pieces.

Squeeze the juice out of the lemon and set aside.

In a blender, add the chopped ginger and turmeric along with the water.

Blend until smooth.

Using a fine mesh strainer or cheesecloth, strain the juice into a glass or container.

Add honey (if desired) and the lemon juice, and stir well.

Serve chilled and enjoy!

Ginger and turmeric are both known for their anti-inflammatory properties and are believed to boost the immune system. Lemon juice adds a refreshing flavor and also provides vitamin C, which is essential for a healthy immune system. Honey can add a touch of sweetness to the juice and also has antibacterial properties. This juice can be consumed regularly to support your overall health and well-being.

5. Vitamin C Powerhouse Juice

Here's a recipe for a Vitamin C Powerhouse Juice:

Ingredients:

2 medium-sized oranges

1 medium-sized grapefruit

1 lemon

1-inch piece of fresh ginger

1 medium-sized carrot

1 medium-sized beetroot

Instructions:

Peel the oranges, grapefruit and lemon, and cut them into small pieces. Remove the seeds.

Peel and grate the ginger.

Wash the carrot and beetroot and chop them into small pieces.

Put all the ingredients into a juicer and blend until smooth.

Pour the juice into a glass and serve immediately.

This juice is packed with vitamin C, which is essential for a healthy immune system, and antioxidants that help fight against free radicals. It's a refreshing and delicious way to get your daily dose of vitamins and minerals. Enjoy!

6. Super Green Juice

Here's a recipe for making this delicious juice:

Ingredients:

2 cups of spinach leaves

1 cucumber

1 lemon

1 green apple

1 inch of fresh ginger root

1/2 teaspoon of turmeric powder

1/2 teaspoon of honey (optional)

Instructions:

Wash all the ingredients thoroughly.

Cut the cucumber, lemon, and apple into small pieces.

Peel the ginger root and cut it into small pieces.

Put all the ingredients into a blender and blend until smooth.

If desired, add honey to sweeten the juice.

Pour the juice into a glass and serve immediately.

This Super Green Cold and Flu Juice is packed with nutrients that can help strengthen your immune system, fight inflammation, and alleviate cold and flu symptoms. Spinach is a good source of vitamins A and C, which are both important for immune function. Cucumber is high in water and can help keep you hydrated, while also providing vitamin K and antioxidants. Lemon is a good source of vitamin C and has antibacterial and antiviral properties. Green apple is rich in fiber, vitamins, and antioxidants. Ginger root has anti-inflammatory and pain-relieving properties and can help soothe sore throats and coughs. Finally, turmeric powder has powerful anti-inflammatory and antioxidant effects and can help alleviate symptoms of cold and flu.

7. Cold and Flu Tonic Juice

Cold and flu tonic juice is a healthy and refreshing drink that can help you boost your immune system, fight off infections, and relieve symptoms of the common cold and flu. This juice is packed with immune-boosting vitamins, minerals, and antioxidants that can help your body fight off viruses and bacteria.

Ingredients:

1 small piece of ginger (peeled and chopped)

1 lemon (peeled and sliced)

1 orange (peeled and sliced)

1 medium-sized carrot (peeled and chopped)

2-3 cloves of garlic (peeled and chopped)

1-2 tablespoons of honey (optional)

1/4 teaspoon of turmeric (optional)

1/4 teaspoon of cayenne pepper (optional)

1/4 teaspoon of black pepper (optional)

1/2 cup of water

Instructions:

Wash and chop all the ingredients.

Put the ginger, lemon, orange, carrot, and garlic into a blender.

Add water to the blender and blend until smooth.

If desired, add honey, turmeric, cayenne pepper, and black pepper to the juice and blend again.

Pour the juice into a glass and drink immediately.

Benefits:

Ginger contains compounds that have anti-inflammatory and antioxidant properties. It can help to reduce inflammation and pain in the body and boost the immune system.

Lemon is a good source of vitamin C, which is an essential nutrient for the immune system. Vitamin C can help to boost the production of white blood cells, which are the cells that fight off infections.

Orange is also rich in vitamin C, as well as other vitamins and minerals that are important for immune function, such as vitamin A, folate, and potassium.

Carrot is a good source of beta-carotene, which is a precursor to vitamin A. Vitamin A is important for the immune system and can help to protect the body against infections.

Garlic contains compounds that have antibacterial and antiviral properties. It can help to boost the immune system and fight off infections.

Honey has antibacterial and anti-inflammatory properties and can help to soothe sore throats and coughs.

Turmeric contains a compound called curcumin, which has anti-inflammatory and antioxidant properties. It can help to reduce inflammation in the body and boost the immune system.

Cayenne pepper contains a compound called capsaicin, which can help to reduce pain and inflammation in the body.

Black pepper contains a compound called piperine, which can help to increase the absorption of other nutrients in the body.

8. Immune-Boosting Green Juice

Here's a recipe for an immune-boosting green juice:

Ingredients:

2 cups spinach

2 cups kale

2 medium cucumbers

2 medium green apples

1/2 lemon, peeled

1-inch piece of ginger

1/4 teaspoon turmeric powder

Instructions:

Wash all the ingredients well.

Chop the kale, spinach, and cucumbers into smaller pieces.

Cut the apples into wedges, removing the core and seeds.

Peel the lemon and ginger.

Add all the ingredients to a juicer and blend until smooth.

Serve immediately and enjoy!

This juice is packed with vitamins, minerals, and antioxidants that can help boost your immune system. Spinach and kale are rich in vitamins A and C, which can help support immune function. Cucumbers are a good source of vitamin K, which is important for healthy blood clotting, and they also contain antioxidants that can help reduce inflammation. Green apples add natural sweetness to the juice and are high in vitamin C. Lemon and ginger add a refreshing zing to the juice and also contain antioxidants that can help protect against disease. Turmeric powder is known for its anti-inflammatory properties and can also help support immune function.

9. Berry and Beet Juice

Berry and Beet cold and flu juice is a delicious and nutritious juice recipe that can help boost your immune system and provide relief from cold and flu symptoms. Here's how to make it:

Ingredients:

1 medium beetroot

1 cup mixed berries (e.g. blueberries, raspberries, blackberries)

1 medium orange, peeled

1-inch piece of ginger, peeled

1-2 cups water (depending on desired consistency)

Honey (optional)

Instructions:

Wash the beetroot and cut it into small pieces.

Add the beetroot, mixed berries, orange, and ginger to a juicer or blender and blend until smooth.

Add water to the mixture until you reach your desired consistency. If the juice is too tart, you can add honey to taste.

Pour the juice into glasses and enjoy immediately.

This juice is packed with vitamins, antioxidants, and anti-inflammatory compounds that can help strengthen your immune system and fight off cold and flu symptoms. Beets are rich in vitamin C and antioxidants, while berries are high in vitamin C and flavonoids. Oranges are another excellent source of vitamin C, and ginger has natural anti-inflammatory properties that can help relieve sore throats and other cold and flu symptoms.

10. Citrus and Carrot Juice

The vitamin C in citrus fruits like oranges and lemons can help boost your immune system, while the beta-carotene in carrots can help keep your skin healthy and aid in respiratory health.

Here is a simple recipe for a citrus and carrot cold and flu juice:

Ingredients:

3 carrots, peeled and chopped

2 oranges, peeled and segmented

1 lemon, peeled and segmented

1-inch piece of ginger, peeled and chopped

1/2 cup of water

Instructions:

Add the chopped carrots, oranges, lemon, and ginger to a blender or juicer.

Blend until the mixture is smooth.

Add the water and blend again until well combined.

Pour the juice into a glass and serve immediately.

You can also experiment with different citrus fruits, such as grapefruit or tangerines, and add other ingredients like turmeric or honey to taste. Just be sure to wash all your ingredients thoroughly before preparing your juice.

11. Carrot and Ginger Juice

Ingredients:

4 medium-sized carrots, peeled and chopped

1-inch piece of fresh ginger, peeled and chopped

1/2 lemon, juiced

1 tablespoon honey (optional)

1 cup cold water

Ice cubes (optional)

Instructions:

Wash, peel, and chop the carrots into small pieces.

Peel and chop the ginger into small pieces.

In a blender, add the chopped carrots and ginger.

Add the lemon juice, honey (if using), and cold water.

Blend on high speed for 1-2 minutes or until the mixture becomes smooth.

Taste the juice and adjust the sweetness with more honey, if needed.

Pour the juice into a glass and serve over ice cubes, if desired.

Enjoy your delicious and healthy carrot and ginger cold and flu juice!

Note: This recipe makes about 2 servings. You can store any leftovers in an airtight container in the refrigerator for up to max. 24-48 hours. Shake well before drinking.

12. Apple and Cranberry Juice

Ingredients:

1 cup fresh cranberries

2 apples, cored and chopped

1-inch piece of fresh ginger, peeled

1 lemon, juiced

2 cups of water

Instructions:

Rinse the cranberries and set aside.

Peel the ginger and chop it into small pieces.

Juice the lemon and set aside.

Core and chop the apples into small pieces.

Add the water, cranberries, chopped apples, and ginger to a blender.

Blend until smooth.

Strain the mixture through a fine-mesh sieve to remove any large particles.

Add the lemon juice to the strained juice and stir to combine.

Pour the juice into a glass and serve.

This juice is packed with vitamin C, antioxidants, and anti-inflammatory compounds that can help boost the immune system and alleviate cold and flu symptoms. It's also a great way to stay hydrated and nourished when you're feeling under the weather. Enjoy!

13. Green Detox Juice

Here's a simple recipe for a delicious and nutritious green detox juice:

Ingredients:

2 green apples, cored and sliced

1 cucumber, chopped

1 handful of spinach

1/2 lemon, juiced

1-inch piece of ginger, peeled and grated

1 cup of water

Instructions:

Wash and prepare all the ingredients as required.

Add the green apples, cucumber, spinach, lemon juice, and ginger to a blender.

Pour in the water and blend all the ingredients until smooth.

Taste and adjust the flavors as needed by adding more lemon juice or ginger.

Pour the juice into a glass and serve chilled.

Enjoy your delicious and healthy green detox juice!

14. Spicy Ginger Juice

Here's a recipe for Spicy Ginger Juice for Cold and Flu:

Ingredients:

2 large oranges, peeled

2 medium carrots, peeled

1 medium apple, cored

1-inch piece of fresh ginger, peeled

1/4 teaspoon cayenne pepper

1/4 teaspoon turmeric powder

1/4 teaspoon honey (optional)

Ice cubes (optional)

Instructions:

Wash all the ingredients thoroughly.

Cut the oranges, carrots, and apple into small pieces that will fit into your juicer.

Cut the ginger into small pieces.

Juice all the ingredients except for the cayenne pepper and turmeric powder.

Stir in the cayenne pepper and turmeric powder.

Taste the juice and add honey if desired.

Pour the juice into a glass filled with ice cubes (optional) and enjoy!

This juice is packed with vitamin C from the oranges, beta-carotene from the carrots, and anti-inflammatory properties from the ginger, turmeric, and cayenne pepper. It's a great way to boost your immune system and fight off colds and flu.

15. Cold Buster Juice

Cold Buster Juice is a healthy and delicious juice that can help alleviate the symptoms of the common cold and boost your immune system. It is a combination of fruits and vegetables that are rich in vitamin C, antioxidants, and other nutrients that help fight off infections and reduce inflammation. This juice is perfect for those who want to stay healthy during the cold and flu season.

Here's how you can make Cold Buster Juice at home:

Ingredients:

2 oranges

2 carrots

1 lemon

1 ginger root

1 apple

1/2 cup of water

Optional: 1-2 tablespoons of honey for sweetness

Instructions:

Wash all the fruits and vegetables thoroughly.

Peel the oranges and lemon and remove the seeds from the apple.

Cut the oranges, carrots, lemon, and apple into small pieces.

Cut a small piece of ginger root and peel off the skin.

Add all the ingredients into a blender or juicer.

Add 1/2 cup of water and blend until smooth.

Taste the juice and add honey if needed for sweetness.

Pour the juice into a glass and enjoy.

Ginger root is a natural anti-inflammatory and anti-bacterial agent that helps boost the immune system and relieve symptoms of cold and flu. It also helps soothe sore throats and reduce nausea. Honey is a natural sweetener that also has antibacterial properties, making it a perfect addition to Cold Buster Juice.

Cold Buster Juice is an excellent source of vitamin C, which is a powerful antioxidant that helps protect your immune system against infections. Oranges, lemon, and apple are all rich in vitamin C and other essential nutrients like fiber and potassium, which help improve digestion and regulate blood pressure. Carrots are also a great source of beta-carotene, which converts into vitamin A in the body and helps maintain healthy skin and eyes.

Serve and Enjoy!

CHAPTER 4

Juicing for Prevention: How to Stay Healthy During Cold and Flu Season

4.1 Tips for Maintaining a Healthy Immune System

Maintaining a healthy immune system is essential to staying healthy and avoiding illnesses. The immune system is responsible for protecting the body against harmful substances, including bacteria, viruses, and other pathogens. A healthy immune system can also help to prevent chronic diseases, such as cancer and autoimmune disorders.

Here are some tips for maintaining a healthy immune system:

1. **Eat a Healthy Diet**: Eating a diet that is rich in fruits, vegetables, whole grains, and lean protein can help to keep your immune system healthy. These foods contain essential vitamins, minerals, and antioxidants that can help to boost your immune system and keep it functioning properly.

2. **Stay Hydrated**: Drinking enough water is important for maintaining a healthy immune system. Water helps to flush out toxins and waste products from the body, which can help to keep your immune system functioning at its best.

3. **Get Enough Sleep**: Getting enough sleep is essential for a healthy immune system. During sleep, the body repairs and regenerates cells, including immune cells. Aim to get at least 7-8 hours of sleep each night to support your immune system.

4. **Avoid Smoking and Limit Alcohol**: Smoking can weaken the immune system and increase the risk of infections. Alcohol can also have a negative impact on the immune system, so it's important to limit your alcohol intake.

5. **Wash Your Hands**: Proper hand hygiene is essential for preventing the spread of infections.

Wash your hands frequently with soap and water for at least 20 seconds, especially after being in public spaces or around people who are sick.

6. **Get Vaccinated**: Vaccines can help to prevent infectious diseases and boost the immune system. Talk to your healthcare provider about the recommended vaccines for your age and health status.

7. **Stay Connected with Others**: Social connections can have a positive impact on mental health and can also boost the immune system. Stay connected with friends and family members, even if it's just through phone or video calls.

4.2 Building a Strong Foundation for a Healthy Body

A strong foundation for a healthy body requires a holistic approach that incorporates various aspects of a person's life. It involves adopting healthy lifestyle habits that promote physical, mental, and emotional well-being. The following are some ways to build a strong foundation for a healthy body:

Exercise regularly: Exercise is important for overall health and can also help to boost your immune system. Regular exercise can improve circulation, reduce inflammation, and help to flush out toxins from the body. Exercise is essential for maintaining a healthy body. It helps to build strength, endurance, and flexibility, improve cardiovascular health, and boost mood. It is recommended that adults engage in at least 150 minutes of moderate-intensity aerobic activity or 75 minutes of vigorous-intensity aerobic activity per week.

Eat a healthy diet: A healthy diet is crucial for maintaining a healthy body. It should include a variety of nutrient-dense foods such as fruits, vegetables, whole grains, lean proteins, and healthy fats. Limiting processed foods, added sugars, and saturated fats can also improve overall health.

Manage stress: Chronic stress can have negative effects on the body, including increasing the risk of chronic diseases. It is essential to find healthy ways to manage stress such as meditation, yoga, or deep breathing exercises.

Maintain a healthy weight: Being overweight or obese can increase the risk of chronic diseases such as heart disease, diabetes, and certain cancers. Maintaining a healthy weight through a combination of healthy eating habits and regular exercise can improve overall health.

Get enough sleep: Sleep is critical for physical and mental health. It helps the body to repair and regenerate, improves mood and cognitive function, and boosts immunity. Adults should aim for 7-8 hours of sleep per night.

Avoid harmful habits: Smoking, excessive alcohol consumption, and drug use can have negative effects on the body. Quitting smoking, limiting alcohol consumption, and avoiding drug use can improve overall health and reduce the risk of chronic diseases.

Regular check-ups: Regular check-ups with a healthcare provider can help identify and manage health issues early on. It is recommended that adults receive regular health screenings such as blood pressure, cholesterol, and cancer screenings.

4.3 Making Juicing a Part of Your Daily Routine

Juicing has become a popular trend in recent years as people have become more health-conscious and interested in living a healthier lifestyle. Juicing involves extracting the juice from fruits and vegetables using a juicer or blender, providing a concentrated dose of nutrients and vitamins that can be quickly absorbed by the body. Making juicing a part of your daily routine can offer numerous health benefits, including improved digestion, enhanced immune system, increased energy levels, and weight loss. Here are some tips for making juicing a part of your daily routine.

Start Small

If you're new to juicing, it's best to start small and gradually increase your intake. Begin with one or two glasses of juice per day and slowly increase the amount over time. This will help your body adjust to the new routine and prevent any digestive discomfort.

Choose the Right Equipment

Invest in a good quality juicer or blender to ensure that you get the most out of your fruits and vegetables. Centrifugal juicers are the most common type of juicer, but they may not be the best choice for leafy greens and herbs. Masticating juicers are better suited for these types of produce as they extract more juice and preserve more nutrients.

Plan Your Juicing

Planning is key to making juicing a part of your daily routine. Decide when you will juice and what ingredients you will use. Consider preparing your ingredients the night before to save time in the morning. You can also make larger batches of juice and store them in the fridge for later.

Experiment with Ingredients

One of the great things about juicing is that you can experiment with different fruits and vegetables to find the flavors that you like. Don't be afraid to mix and match ingredients to create your own unique recipes. You can also add herbs, spices, and superfoods like chia seeds, hemp seeds, and spirulina for an extra boost of nutrition.

Make It Fun

Juicing doesn't have to be a chore. Make it a fun activity by involving your family or friends. Try creating different recipes together or have a juicing party where everyone brings their own ingredients to share. You can also try juicing challenges where you set goals and track your progress.

Be Consistent

Consistency is key when it comes to making juicing a part of your daily routine. Try to juice at the same time every day, whether it's in the morning, afternoon, or evening. This will help you establish a routine and make it easier to stick to.

Incorporate Juicing into Your Diet

Juicing shouldn't replace whole fruits and vegetables in your diet, but it can be a great supplement. Try to incorporate juicing into your diet by using it as a snack or meal replacement. You can also add juice to smoothies, oatmeal, or yogurt for an extra boost of nutrition.

CHAPTER 5

JUICING FOR RECOVERY: HOW TO GET BACK ON YOUR FEET FASTER

5.1 The Importance of Rest and Recovery

Rest and recovery are crucial elements for managing and recovering from cold and flu. Cold and flu are viral infections that can affect anyone, and they are highly contagious. The symptoms of cold and flu can make people feel terrible and can often leave them feeling fatigued and weak. This is where rest and recovery come in, as they can help the body recover from the infection.

Rest is essential for cold and flu recovery because it helps the body conserve energy that it needs to fight the infection. When you rest, you reduce the amount of energy your body uses for other activities like moving around or digesting food. This way, your body can focus its energy on fighting the virus.

Additionally, rest helps the body recover by allowing the immune system to work effectively.

When you sleep or rest, your body releases certain hormones, such as growth hormone and cortisol, that help support the immune system. These hormones promote the production of white blood cells and antibodies, which are essential for fighting infections.

Another important aspect of rest is that it helps reduce stress levels. Stress can weaken the immune system and make it more difficult for the body to fight off infections. By resting and reducing stress levels, you give your body a chance to heal and recover more quickly.

Recovery from cold and flu also requires proper nutrition and hydration. When you have a cold or flu, your body uses up a lot of energy and nutrients to fight the infection. It is essential to consume a balanced diet that provides enough energy and nutrients to support the immune system. Foods rich in vitamins and minerals, such as fruits, vegetables, and lean proteins, can help provide the necessary nutrients.

Drinking plenty of fluids is also important during recovery. Fluids help keep the body hydrated, which is necessary for maintaining proper immune function. Water, herbal tea, and soup are all excellent options for staying hydrated.

In addition to rest and proper nutrition, recovery from cold and flu also requires avoiding physical exertion and exposure to other sick people. Physical exertion can drain the body of energy and make it more difficult for the immune system to fight off the infection. Exposure to other sick people can increase the risk of catching another infection, which can prolong the recovery process.

In conclusion, rest and recovery are essential for managing and recovering from cold and flu. Rest helps conserve energy, promote immune system function, and reduce stress levels, while proper nutrition and hydration provide the necessary nutrients to support the immune system. To recover from cold and flu, it is also important to avoid physical exertion and exposure to other sick people. By following these guidelines, you can help your body recover more quickly and get back to your daily activities.

Rest and Recovery

for Overall Well-being and Success

Rest and recovery are essential aspects of maintaining good health and achieving optimal performance in any aspect of life. Whether you are an athlete, a student, stay at home or a working professional, giving your body and mind sufficient time to rest and recover can make a significant difference in your overall well-being and success.

Here are some key reasons why rest and recovery are important:

Reduces the risk of injury: Taking regular breaks and allowing your body to recover after intense physical activity can reduce the risk of injury. Without adequate rest, your body may become overworked and fatigued, making it more prone to injury.

Improves performance: Rest and recovery are critical for improving performance. When you give your body enough time to rest and recover, you allow your muscles to repair and rebuild themselves, which can lead to increased strength, endurance, and overall performance.

Enhances mental health: Rest and recovery are not just important for physical health, but also for mental health. Taking time off to relax and recharge can help reduce stress levels, improve mood, and enhance cognitive function.

Boosts immunity: Sleep and rest are essential for boosting the immune system. Studies have shown that lack of sleep can weaken the immune system, making you more susceptible to illness and disease.

Improves sleep quality: Adequate rest and recovery can improve the quality of your sleep, which is essential for good health. Poor sleep quality can lead to a variety of health problems, including obesity, diabetes, and heart disease.

Helps prevent burnout: Taking regular breaks and giving your body and mind sufficient time to rest can help prevent burnout. Burnout is a state of emotional, physical, and mental exhaustion that can occur when you are under constant stress and pressure.

Improves overall well-being: Rest and recovery are essential for maintaining overall health and well-being. When you prioritize rest and recovery, you are giving your body the time it needs to heal, repair, and rejuvenate, which can help you feel better and perform better in all areas of your life.

There are many ways to incorporate rest and recovery into your daily routine. Some strategies include getting enough sleep each night, taking regular breaks throughout the day, practicing relaxation techniques such as meditation or yoga, and engaging in low-impact activities such as walking or swimming.

In conclusion, rest and recovery are essential for maintaining good health and achieving optimal performance. By prioritizing rest and recovery, you can reduce the risk of injury, improve performance, enhance mental health, boost immunity, improve sleep quality, prevent burnout, and improve overall well-being. So, take the time to rest and recover – your body and mind will thank you for it.

5.2 Nutrient-Dense Juices to Support Your Recovery

When you're feeling under the weather with a cold or flu, it can be challenging to muster up the energy to cook or even chew food. However, it's essential to nourish your body with nutrients to aid in your recovery. One effective way to do this is by drinking nutrient-dense juices. Here are some juices that can help support your cold and flu recovery:

Orange juice: Orange juice is a classic cold-fighting juice that is packed with vitamin C, which is essential for strengthening the immune system.

It also contains folate, potassium, and thiamine, which can help reduce inflammation and provide energy. However, it's important to note that store-bought orange juice often has added sugars and preservatives, so it's best to make your own fresh juice.

Pineapple juice: Pineapple juice contains bromelain, which is an enzyme that has anti-inflammatory properties that can help reduce swelling and inflammation in the sinuses and throat. It also contains vitamin C, manganese, and potassium, which can help boost the immune system and provide energy.

Carrot juice: Carrot juice is rich in beta-carotene, which is converted into vitamin A in the body. Vitamin A is essential for maintaining healthy mucous membranes in the nose and throat, which can help prevent infection. Carrot juice also contains vitamin C, potassium, and folate, which can help boost the immune system and provide energy. Carrot juice is also rich in other antioxidants, such as vitamin C and E, which can help reduce inflammation and support overall health.

Ginger juice: Ginger has been used for centuries as a natural remedy for colds and flu. Juicing ginger can help you consume higher amounts of this beneficial root.

Ginger is a natural anti-inflammatory and antibacterial agent that can help reduce inflammation and fight off infection. It has powerful anti-inflammatory and antioxidant properties that can help reduce inflammation, ease congestion, and relieve nausea Ginger juice also contains gingerol, which is an antioxidant that can help boost the immune system. It's best to make your own fresh ginger juice by blending or juicing fresh ginger root with a little bit of water. You can also add it to other juices for an extra boost of flavor and health benefits.

Beet juice: Beet juice is a good source of iron, which is essential for maintaining healthy red blood cells that transport oxygen throughout the body. It also contains vitamin C, potassium, and folate, which can help boost the immune system and provide energy. Beets are rich in nitrates, which your body converts to nitric oxide. Nitric oxide is a vasodilator that can help improve blood flow, oxygenation in the body and also reduce inflammation.

Turmeric juice: Turmeric contains curcumin, which is a natural anti-inflammatory and antioxidant that can help reduce inflammation and fight off infection. Turmeric juice also contains vitamin C, potassium, and iron, which can help boost the immune system and provide energy. It's best to make your own fresh turmeric juice by blending or juicing fresh turmeric root with a little bit of water.

Citrus Juices

Citrus fruits are packed with vitamin C, which is known for its immune-boosting properties. Juices made with oranges, grapefruits, lemons, limes, and other citrus fruits can help increase your intake of this essential vitamin. Vitamin C is also an antioxidant that can help reduce inflammation and protect your cells from damage caused by free radicals.

Kale Juice

Kale is a nutrient-dense leafy green that's rich in vitamins A, C, and K, as well as calcium, iron, and other minerals. Juicing kale can help you consume more of these important nutrients, which can help support your immune system, reduce inflammation, and promote overall health.

When making nutrient-dense juices for cold and flu recovery, it's essential to use fresh, organic fruits and vegetables that are free of pesticides and other harmful chemicals. It's also important to avoid adding extra sugar or other additives to your juices, as these can reduce the overall health benefits of the juice. You can also experiment with different combinations of fruits, vegetables, and spices to find the flavors and nutrients that work best for you. Drinking nutrient-dense juices can be an excellent way to support your cold and flu recovery while providing your body with the nutrients it needs to heal.

5.3 Foods to Avoid While Recovering

When you're recovering from a cold or flu, what you eat can have a significant impact on how quickly you recover. Certain foods can provide much-needed nutrients and support your immune system, while others can actually make your symptoms worse.

Here are some of the foods to avoid while recovering from a cold or flu.

Sugary Foods and Drinks

Sugary foods and drinks can suppress your immune system, making it harder for your body to fight off the infection. Additionally, they can cause inflammation and make symptoms like sore throat and cough worse. It's best to avoid sugary foods and drinks like candy, soda, and processed baked goods while recovering from a cold or flu.

Dairy Products

Dairy products like milk, cheese, and ice cream can thicken mucus, making it harder to clear your airways. This can exacerbate symptoms like congestion and cough. If you're experiencing these symptoms, it's best to avoid dairy products or choose low-fat options like skim milk or yogurt.

Fried and Greasy Foods

Fried and greasy foods can be hard to digest, which can take energy away from your immune system and slow down the healing process. Additionally, they can cause inflammation and worsen symptoms like headache and fatigue. Stick to light and easily digestible foods like broths, soups, and steamed vegetables while recovering from a cold or flu.

Alcohol and Caffeine

Alcohol and caffeine can dehydrate you, which can make your symptoms worse and slow down the healing process. Additionally, they can interfere with sleep, which is important for allowing your body to rest and recover. It's best to avoid alcohol and caffeine while recovering from a cold or flu.

Spicy Foods

Spicy foods can irritate your throat and make symptoms like cough and sore throat worse. Additionally, they can cause indigestion and heartburn, which can be uncomfortable while you're already feeling unwell. It's best to avoid spicy foods like hot sauce, chili peppers, and curry while recovering from a cold or flu.

Processed Foods

Processed foods are often high in salt, preservatives, and additives, which can be hard on your body when you're already feeling unwell. Additionally, they're often low in nutrients and can't provide the vitamins and minerals your body needs to recover. Stick to whole, nutrient-dense foods like fruits, vegetables, and lean proteins while recovering from a cold or flu.

Large Meals

Large meals can be hard on your digestive system, which can take energy away from your immune system and slow down the healing process. Additionally, they can cause indigestion and bloating, which can be uncomfortable while you're already feeling unwell. Stick to small, frequent meals and snacks to keep your energy levels up while recovering from a cold or flu.

Overall, while recovering from a cold or flu, it's important to avoid sugary foods and drinks, dairy products, fried and greasy foods, alcohol and caffeine, spicy foods, processed foods, and large meals. Instead, choose light, nutrient-dense foods that can provide the vitamins and minerals your body needs to recover. Don't forget to stay hydrated and get plenty of rest to support your body's natural healing processes.

CONCLUSION

Juicing is the process of extracting juice from fruits and vegetables using a juicer. This juice contains a variety of vitamins, minerals, antioxidants, and enzymes that are beneficial for the body. Juicing has gained popularity in recent years as a way to boost overall health and wellness, as well as for its potential to help with specific health concerns like cold and flu.

Cold and flu are common illnesses that affect millions of people worldwide every year. These illnesses are caused by viruses that attack the respiratory system, leading to symptoms such as cough, sore throat, runny nose, and fever. There are several ways to manage symptoms and boost the immune system to help fight off the viruses.

One of the great ways to support the immune system during cold and flu is through juicing.

Some of the benefits of juicing for cold and flu:

High in Vitamin C: Fruits and vegetables such as oranges, lemons, grapefruits, strawberries, and bell peppers are rich in vitamin C, which is a powerful antioxidant that helps boost the immune system.

Juicing these fruits and vegetables can provide a concentrated dose of vitamin C, which can help fight off the viruses causing cold and flu.

Anti-inflammatory: Many fruits and vegetables contain anti-inflammatory compounds that can help reduce inflammation in the body, which is often present during cold and flu. Examples of anti-inflammatory compounds found in fruits and vegetables include bromelain (found in pineapple), curcumin (found in turmeric), and gingerols (found in ginger).

Hydration: Staying hydrated is important during cold and flu, as it can help loosen mucus and relieve congestion. Juicing fruits and vegetables that are high in water content, such as cucumber, celery, and watermelon, can help keep the body hydrated and support the respiratory system.

Digestive Support: Cold and flu can often affect the digestive system, leading to nausea, diarrhea, and vomiting. Juicing fruits and vegetables that are high in fiber, such as apples, pears, and leafy greens, can help support the digestive system and promote healthy bowel movements.

Improved Nutrient Absorption: Juicing can help improve the absorption of nutrients from fruits and vegetables by breaking down the cell walls of the produce and releasing the nutrients into an easily digestible form.

Increased Energy: Juicing can help increase energy levels by providing a quick boost of vitamins, minerals, and antioxidants that the body needs to function properly.

Detoxification: Juicing can help support the body's natural detoxification process by providing the liver and kidneys with the nutrients they need to eliminate toxins from the body.

Weight Management: Juicing can be a helpful tool for weight management, as it can provide a low-calorie, nutrient-dense source of energy that can help support a healthy diet and lifestyle.

When juicing for cold and flu, it's important to choose fruits and vegetables that are high in vitamin C, anti-inflammatory compounds, and water content. Some great options include oranges, lemons, grapefruits, strawberries, bell peppers, pineapple, turmeric, ginger, cucumber, celery, watermelon, apples, pears, and leafy greens.

It's also important to take care of yourself by staying hydrated, getting plenty of rest, and eating a well-balanced diet, even when you're not sick.

www.ingramcontent.com/pod-product-compliance
Lightning Source LLC
Chambersburg PA
CBHW071058250726
48662CB00019B/1251